Whole Foods vs.

Processed Foods

How to create a healthy relationship with food

By PROSENCE

publisher for any reparation, damages, or monetary loss due to the information herein, either directly or indirectly.

Respective authors own all copyrights not held by the publisher.

The information herein is offered for informational purposes solely, and is universal as so. The presentation of the information is without contract or any type of guarantee assurance.

The trademarks that are used are without any consent, and the publication of the trademark is without permission or backing by the trademark owner. All trademarks and brands within this book are for clarifying purposes only and are the owned by the owners themselves, not affiliated with this document.

ABOUT PROSENCE

Our Mission

We are dedicated to guiding, motivating and providing the tools necessary to transform people into the best version of themselves. Our goal is to empower men and women across the globe to realize that physical and mental fitness are not a short-term solution, but a lifetime choice, and to actualize what they have come to understand into a daily routine. We invite you to discover this process for yourself as you join us in the exploration of science-based knowledge that can lead to better health, greater fulfillment and astonishing vitality.

Who is Prosence?

Hi, I'm Antonio Mazzotta - certified Fitness Trainer and health enthusiast, and the founder of Prosence. While I don't think I'll ever turn down mom's homemade pasta and pizza, as an Italian living in Switzerland I've built a life dedicated to health and fitness. Now, I want to share the secrets to my success with you.

I got involved in this industry over 7 years ago, and quickly developed a passion for all things health and fitness. I knew right away that this is what I was born to do and haven't looked back. My days are spent developing new routines, training hard and meeting other fitness-minded and health-conscious individuals. I love working with my clients and coaching about weight training, dieting and healthy lifestyle choices. My number one priority is motivating people to achieve any fitness goal they seek. Whether you're looking to lose fat, get stronger, build muscle or just maintain overall health and vitality – Let's reach your goals together!

My team and I work hard to dispel the health and fitness myths and misinformation clogging the Internet today. We're driven by the desire to offer you a safe and manageable yet powerfully effective path to the best health of your life. Prosence is firmly committed to motivating, inspiring, and educating through the sharing of objective, fact-based health and fitness information that is rooted in science. We give you the tools you need to get in great shape and build a lifetime of good health.

Join us - let's work together to maximize your potential and achieve your optimal self while embracing life to the fullest!

Learn more on our website: www.prosencefitness.com, blog and keep up with the daily education and motivation by liking us on Twitter, Facebook & Instagram @prosencefitness.

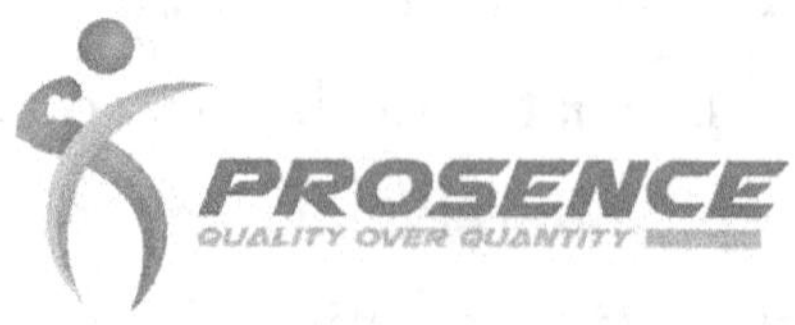

Table of Contents

Introduction

If you've ever googled the proper way to manage your diet, there's a good chance you've come across the terms "whole food" and "processed food". There's a lot of hype surrounding these food categories in popular culture and it leads to extreme views on these food categories that can be a bit more harmful than beneficial. Unfortunately the extreme views are often the most common because they're the easiest to grasp onto. In reality an approach that takes more of a middle ground on the consumption of whole and processed foods is best for most people. Behavior change is hard, and most people struggle a lot. Extreme positions make it harder for people with ambition to achieve their goals, making the experience of exercising and dieting become more frustrating than it needs to be.

We here at Prosence are here to help guide you through the definitions of whole and processed foods (they're probably not what you think), inform you of the history of each term, and explain the pros and cons of each as it applies to the diet of a healthy adult.

Is your brain ready to start processing a whole book on this stuff? If so, let's get started.

Chapter 1

Origins of Whole Foods

Whole foods are minimally refined and involve the use of few or no artificial additives. Whole foods are foods that were prepared using natural means without chemical augmentation. Any food that is derived from a plant product can be considered whole food. They are what have been historically consumed by humans for many centuries.

In accordance with Darwin's theory of evolution, most people logically conclude that the foods that have been available to humans for centuries are the ones humans have most biologically adapted to consume. This train of thought supports extreme contemporary diet fads like paleo. Though extreme diets are almost never the answer and often overlook a lot of key details, oversimplifying science, the underlying premise that whole foods aren't bad is generally correct.

Humans have grown and adapted to the consumption of foods in their environment throughout history, but have also done the same with animal products. Because of this, a majority of the popular culture's philosophy behind whole food consumption should apply to animal products.

Because of the cultural pushback against processed foods as a result of views on the obesity epidemic, the term whole food has become a prestigious symbol and useful marketing tool for food companies. In contemporary culture, being labeled as a whole food makes an item seem more desirable, healthy, and trustworthy.

Though whole foods are not per se bad, it is important to note that cultural trends deifying whole foods may be a bit misplaced. Because the category is not inclusive of animal products and foods that have been enhanced in beneficial ways, healthy diets that optimally facilitate the achievement of health goals often require more than just whole foods. Though whole foods do tend to avoid a lot of the pitfalls of their more processed alternatives and are often superior.

Chapter 2

Origins of Processed Foods

Processed foods are food that have been altered on a chemical level and/or have been treated with external additives. Almost any food can become processed if it undergoes the proper treatment, and the ultimate effects of processing a food are based on the methods and/or additives used.

Processed foods were first introduced in the prehistoric era in an attempt to preserve food. By adding things like salt to a food, its decay could be slowed and humans could store their food for longer. This practice supported increased survival rates during harsh periods of winter and facilitated more lucrative commerce throughout history.

Modern methods of processing food were first introduced in the early 19th century when canning food became popularized. This method combined the use of conventional additives like salt with processes that chemically altered food like providing it with a heat treatment. Then once adequately processed, food would be placed in a can to extend its shelf life as long as possible. There are a variety of methods for canning, but the ultimate goal of any canning is to typically make food last as long as possible and maintain as much of its fiber and nutrients for as long as possible. Though early methods involved much health risk, they were eventually refined.

Though earlier methods of processing focused on preventing bacteria from entering food, later methods also involved eliminating bacteria from food. This was introduced with the invention of pasteurization in the late 19th century. An inventor had discovered that heating certain liquids and foods could prevent them from causing illness longer. The introduction of this process allowed for the large scale commercialization of products like milk that typically go bad right away without pasteurization. Given the reduced risks of disease and mortality, some countries made it mandatory for products like milk to become pasteurized.

Though earlier advances and goals of food processing were focused on increasing the well-being of consumers, later methods were introduced for the benefit of food processing and food selling companies. Given the cost saving benefits of storing products in bulk for long periods of time and having them always be in stock, companies began employing more and more methods to preserve food longer. To expand the market of food companies, it became important to preserve products long enough for them to be shipped all over the country, and in cases to other parts of the world. Because of the development of this need, the health advantages of processing food became less and less important to most companies. Though there are still companies that process foods in advantageous ways, a majority do not.

Because of company greed, processed foods ended up developing a bad reputation in contemporary culture. They have become pariahs of the food world and seen as the embodiment of convenience over well-being. Given other choices processed food providers often make with production of their food and their corporate-greed filled over-processing many contribute to decreased health and can negatively affect body composition and well-being. Culturally there has been a recent pushback against the consumption of processed foods in observance of this. But that approach may be an overgeneralization given that not all processed foods are created equally, and realistic healthy dieting often warrants the consumption of some processed foods.

Though it's important to note that some additives, processing methods, and chemical changes to what was once whole food do have deleterious effects, and that the most common methods/additives promote poor health. But given processed food is still food, there are health benefits to consumption that are similar to other foods because certain benefits are inherent to certain elements of food in general.

Chapter 3

How They Affect Your Body

Processed foods can affect the body in a variety of ways, as processing foods can affect the food themselves in different ways. Given there are many different methods and ways to combine different additives with hundreds of foods, to claim there is one absolute effect of consumption would be an overgeneralization. But there are general pros and general cons that tend to be observed when processing food.

Firstly, modern food processing can be very complex. Given so many methods have been introduced throughout history and have proven successful, a large number are utilized together to make processed food last as long as possible while reducing the risk of is causing disease. Ironically, because of the number of methods used and steps in contemporary food processing, the risk of contamination from outside sources is elevated. This may involve non harmful contamination, but may also involve deadly contamination. Though when considering this con, it is important to consider that the act of processing food prevents people from becoming ill on a regular basis, downplaying the concerns about the rarer times contamination occurs. Of course, all methods are different, and some methods can promote illness by decreasing bioavailability of certain micronutrients in processed food (which long term can lead to nutritional deficiencies and unwanted side effects).

Heat related processing of food involves chemical changes to the macronutrients and micronutrients within. Given a majority of processing methods utilize heat in some way, changes to the chemical composition of processed nutrients are very common. Some foods end up with reduced concentrations of certain nutrients post processing, but certain nutrients tend to be more or less receptive to reductions in concentration by processing. For example, the total amount of calcium and zinc in food tends to change a lot less than the amount of thiamin, folic acid, and vitamin B-12. Ultimately though, this just means that more of a food needs to be consumed for the same amount of that micronutrient to be consumed. As an example, if after processing roasted lamb, it has 80% of its original magnesium, consuming other magnesium rich foods in the diet can make up for the discrepancy. Though this can be quite problematic and bothersome for many, given that consuming more food to get more micronutrients often means increasing daily caloric intake and promoting weight gain. But more realistically, it just means that many will consume a similar amount of food and end up absorbing less micronutrients overall than they would have if they'd eaten an unprocessed version of the food.

Another concern for weight management is that consuming less nutrient dense foods may lead to less satiety. Having lower satiety means that an individual will feel less full after eating. The less full an individual feels, the more likely it is they will continue eating. Given psychological factors play significant roles in health behavior change and weight management, having a biological mechanism tell someone when to stop eating is extremely important. Many struggle with weight loss and management as it is, but limiting the usefulness of satiety/feelings of fullness makes the battle much harder.

Satiety is an evolutionarily evolved mechanism for consuming an adequate amount of food each day, but modern food processing practices can accidentally trick this system. Given humans evolved to instinctively base the amount of food consumed off of static properties of food, processed food's atypical properties throw it off. Eating less nutritionally dense food makes the body feel as if it's consuming less calories, though that isn't true. Unfortunately the micronutrient concentrations that get reduced through processing don't yield energy and thus their reduction doesn't lead to an accompanying lower calorie intake.

Certain additives can lead to decreased health when consumed in excessive amounts. Given the nature of most processed food, a majority of additives are used exclusively in excessive amounts to guarantee product longevity. Though additives can be beneficial in that they allow people from all over the world access to food, some of the most common ones like salt can have adverse effects. When chronically over-consumed, salt can lead to increased blood pressure. This increases the likelihood of the disease labeled hypertension. Hypertension can increase strain on the heart and increase the likelihood of a myocardial infarction, more commonly known as a heart attack. Given that about ⅓ of Americans over the age of 18 have hypertension, reducing processed food intake can help.

Some additives are used to increase the marketability or taste of products like sweeteners, flavors, food coloring, and stabilizers. They are often used by companies in various combinations to outsell their competition given the nature of capitalism. All categories contain many potential additives that all have different specific effects.

As discussed earlier, processing foods involves the elimination of certain bacteria. This is done with the intent to prolong food and prevent illness. Though this element of processing food is often well-intentioned, it eliminates bacteria in an almost indiscriminate manner. Research scientists in the 21st century have observed that not all bacteria in the body is harmful. Some bacteria actually facilitate weight management and having a comprehensive internal composition of bacteria in the gut and intestines can be healthy. Consuming bacteria-reduced foods can potentially reduce immune system health, which has the potential to increase the likelihood of disease onset.

Overall though, the detriments of processed foods are heavily linked to the specific methods and additives used. A good number of processed foods contain reasonable amounts of salt, maintain a majority of their micronutrients, and allow millions with access to a variety of foods that can support a healthy lifestyle. Furthermore, issues related to the microbiome (internal concentrations of bacteria in the gut and intestine) can be solved by consuming processed foods and whole foods together. Given the realities of many people's lives it is unreasonable for many to avoid processed foods altogether. This is especially true when considering that some companies succeed by developing more healthful processed food. For a good number of processed products, the pros that accompany their consumption far outweigh the cons. It is easy to lose fat, build muscle, increase strength, and be an elite level athlete while consuming many processed foods, provided the right processed foods are consumed. If a healthy adult shopper purchases a processed food with 10 mg sodium (salt) per serving, then they don't have to worry about any significant negative side effects from that additive. If they purchased a product with 2,000 mg sodium per serving, then the shopper would be at greater risk. Given there is a wide range of available types of processed food and it is almost impossible for most modern humans to avoid encountering, they just have to be smart about which processed food they buy. Chicken in a can is very unlikely to kill someone (though caramel coated chocolate bars are a different story). Limiting oneself to unrealistic standards in food consumption during a diet usually leads to failure and it's a big reason that a lot of people don't succeed in weight loss or management. Though of additional note, some additives have beneficial health effects. For example, many milk products are fortified with vitamin D. This fortification supports the absorption of the micronutrient calcium, making processed/fortified milk more useful in the preservation and promotion of bone health.

Though generally speaking, when looking at processed foods as a whole, bad things are typically observed. Because certain methods of processing food have been advantageous to food providing companies (like the inclusion of monosodium glutamate, otherwise known as MSG), a majority of processed foods share common qualities. Added sugars, typically used to enhance flavor in less favorable processed foods, can actually promote inflammation along with other diseases such as type II diabetes if over-consumed (it should be noted that sugar with similar effects can be found in unprocessed foods, but tends to be in lower concentrations). Though, again, it is important to note that there are many processed foods that are healthy and can lead to positive health outcomes, given fresh slightly processed poultry or beef can be helpful. Those that consume the worst processed foods and do so in consistent excess tend to experience obesity, overeating, poor moods, and cancer at greater rates than their counterparts. By finding and consuming processed foods without additives or processes linked to these outcomes, it is reasonable to assume an individual will be at lower risk.

Most people misunderstand what processed foods actually are and only think of the worst kind of processed food. Processed foods are everywhere, and some are very bad and stereotypical, but others are extremely useful tools for creating the perfect diet. The term processed food is very broad and the effects different processed foods can have on the body reflects that.

Whole foods, in contrast, affect the body similarly but without the effects of additives, reduced bacterial concentrations, or decreased nutrient density. Aside from those things, for the most part, whole food corn will have a similar effect to processed corn (minus whatever was done during processing, which varies depending on how the corn was processed). Because of this, the effects of whole food do vary, but when contrasted to their processed counterparts they do the same thing minus the changes. Whatever effect 14 grams of naturally occurring starch in a potato would have on its consumer will be the same whether processed or not. Each individual component of a food will act as it typically does if it hasn't been modified in a processed food. Whole foods are just foods without the extra or modified elements. The other stuff is still the same.

Chapter 4

Their Relationship Within The Gut

Bacteria in the gut, as mentioned earlier, can have a host of beneficial functions that not only help promote weight management, but assist immune system functions. Consuming processed foods usually has a reductive effect on these bacteria through one of several mechanisms.

Though, of additional concern, emulsifiers that are common to many processed foods may have detrimental effects on the gut. Emulsifiers have the roles of preserving food and making food more appetizing. When emulsifiers are consumed, gut inflammation increases. Inflammation is generally not desired because it can impede regular gut functioning. This can mess with the body's ability to absorb certain nutrients and regulate other important digestive processes given it relates to an unhealthy immune function.

Flora in the gut help strengthen and maintain immune function, and they are supported by whole and unprocessed foods but impeded by processed foods. Because of this, it is important for a variety of foods to be consumed, and though it is okay for diets to have some processed food, it shouldn't comprise 100% of the diet.

Chapter 5

Foods To Eat

Generally, most whole foods are going to be a solid choice. There is nothing inherently wrong with a food being a whole food if consumed before the food item expires (given expiration dates should be shorter than processed foods). As long as whole food is consumed in a balanced diet that meets an individual's macronutrient (protein, carbohydrates, and fat) and micronutrient (vitamins and minerals) needs, then there is no foreseeable harm in consuming it in large amounts.

Though it is important for those whose beliefs and lifestyle choices permit it to consume things like meat (which by default do not fall into the category of a whole food). They provide a number of benefits and are advantageous to consuming for certain vitamins and minerals, as well as the macronutrient protein. Some processed foods are okay, given food can be processed in hundreds of different ways, and things like frozen chicken breasts are almost always okay. Given all dietary journeys are only successful if feasibility is accounted for, it's important for most consumers to permit the consumption of certain processed foods that aren't as bad and can facilitate health goals. Frozen breaded chicken nuggets may not be the best choice, but a regular frozen skinless chicken breast is often going to do far more good for one's health and well-being than bad. A majority of bad things said about processed food consumption are accurate but doesn't reflect all processed products (usually just the worst of the worst). Unfortunately, the worst of the worst make up the majority of processed foods. But the processed foods that aren't that bad are definitely recommended.

When possible, it is usually a good bet to be safe rather than sorry and consume unprocessed foods over processed foods if there is an appropriate substitute for a processed food. As an example, if attempting to build muscle mass and shopping for a product high in the amino acid leucine (a building block of certain proteins that has a significant impact on muscle building), and only processed meats can be found, it's probably not a wise idea to substitute the meat with carrots. If searching and both processed and unprocessed meats are found, it's usually best to take the unprocessed. Though it is also important to keep in mind that some processed foods are beneficial given their additives. As mentioned earlier, vitamin D fortified milk can be very beneficial given it facilitates the absorption of calcium and can promote increased bone mineral density (which can save an individual from a lot of complications later down the road).

Overall, the best goal is to always consume a balanced diet and prioritize whole foods and unprocessed foods more than processed foods. And when selecting from processed foods it is best to pick those that are less processed over more processed. Consuming processed foods is okay if priorities are in order and the processed foods have a specific dietary function like helping meet protein needs.

Chapter 6

Foods To Avoid

Foods that are highly processed and contain large amounts of certain additives should be avoided. As mentioned earlier MSG, salt, and sugar are common additives in processed food. They promote negative health outcomes if over-consumed and should be scanned for when selecting a food to purchase.

Salt and sugar alone aren't very bad. If consumed in reasonable amounts they can promote a perfectly healthy diet. But because a majority of processed foods contain exorbitant amounts of both it's very common for them to be over-consumed in the modern diet. The American Heart Association recommends that a maximum of 2,300 mg of salt be consumed each day, though less is generally better. It is important to pick low salt foods when possible to avoid exceeding this value and aim for a much lower one. This can be challenging for those who eat primarily processed foods, but not impossible.

The American Heart Association also recommends that men consume a maximum of 9 tsp of sugar per day and that women consume a maximum of 6 tsp of sugar per day. It is extremely easy to exceed these values so it is important to select foods that are lower in sugar and higher in fiber. It is important to note that carbohydrates are still a very necessary component of a well-balanced diet and should still make up a majority of an individual's daily calories. Though the carbohydrates consumed should be regulated so that a minimal amount come from sugar. It is possible to have a high carbohydrate diet without an excess of sugar consumption. Given the rising rates of type II diabetes it is important for individuals to act preemptively and limit sugar consumption.

MSG is never a good thing. It has been linked to metabolic disease, obesity, and almost every other imaginable negative health outcome. It is used as a food preservative and flavor enhancer in certain cultures but does not come with any significant health benefits. It should be avoided at all costs.

For the most part, avoiding food requires the avoidance of foods high in certain elements like salt or sugar, and not the avoidance of those elements altogether. Salt and sugar are fine if consumed in moderation. Though there are things like MSG that should be avoided completely whenever possible. Another item that falls into this category is trans-saturated fat, otherwise known as trans-fat. In the US this can no longer exist within food other than in trace amounts given its extremely negative effects, so it isn't something most individuals have to worry about looking out for. But it is very bad so it is worth mentioning that it should be avoided at all costs if ever encountered.

Chapter 7

Frequently Asked Questions

Are there any benefits to consuming processed food over whole foods? It seems like whole foods is generally superior if it's reasonable to consume it and available.

Yes, there are in some cases, but it depends on the specific food and situation. If availability or cost is an issue, it is typically far better for an individual to consume processed foods to meet their macronutritional and micronutritional needs than to under-consume by not eating anything at all. So much value is placed on the differences between processed and whole foods in modern culture that it becomes easy to forget that processed foods are food as well. But of course when selecting processed food as with any food, those that are more micronutritionally dense and macronutritionally appropriate should be prioritized. Since the quality of a processed food can vary from 'pretty good' to 'completely terrible' the inclusion of processed foods doesn't have to be that detrimental to health if it's necessary for financial or practical reasons.

Furthermore, behavior change is hard for most people. If someone struggles to stick to a diet, maintaining a solid amount of processed food can help an individual succeed with their behavior change. The typical rule of thumb usually thrown around in the nutrition industry is about 80-90% of calories consumed should come from foods that are very healthful and goal oriented, but the other 10-20% can come from whatever helps someone maintain their diet. This isn't a tool that everyone needs to use as some people are fine with never eating processed foods or only minimal amounts, but for those that have difficulty giving up foods it can be a golden ticket. It's better to have a 90% perfect diet than make things too hard, give up, and go back to a 0% perfect diet. This is especially true if considering that processed foods don't have to be evil, they're still food and the right processed food choices can be okay.

Where can I find whole foods? Processed foods are everywhere, but I just wouldn't know where to go to get something organic.

Given recent cultural trends, many markets have been popping up throughout the world in an attempt to answer this very question. One of the most common is Whole Foods Market, which often has a wide selection of whole foods, and aims to have a health-first operation.

If large stores markets aren't an option, local farmer's markets are a choice for many. They pop up multiple times per year all throughout the world. The largest benefit of purchasing whole food goods from a local farmer's market is that it supports the farm(s) contributing. The more they are supported, the more they can produce long term. If they become more successful, their operations can grow and it will be slightly more commonplace to see whole foods around their local community.

Are there any quick tips to tell if a food is processed or not?

Usually it's actually pretty simple! All someone needs to do is find the ingredients list and check how many items there are. If the list is really long, it's likely processed (but not definitely). If the list is really short with only a few basic non-sciency sounding items, it's likely unprocessed (but not definitely). It's not a guaranteed method but it can help anyone briefly check an item and with a high degree of confidence guess which the food item is.

I have a chronic disease, does this advice apply to me?

If you have a chronic disease, do not take nutrition advice from any source other than a personal Registered Dietician who is able to provide you with a personalized plan. Because of the complexities of food, recommendations and advice that may benefit healthy individuals may be harmful to an individual with a chronic disease.

Conclusion

I hope that this food guide will in some way serve to provide all of you out there with the foundation for future success. It can be hard to accomplish your goals if your diet isn't on point. Every little thing you do will count and influence you physiologically, psychologically, or both. Which is why it's important to have as informed a mind as possible when making food choices.

Seeing as we've reached the end of our journey, it's important that you use the information you've learned here to shape your diet, your dream body, and your grocery list. Whatever foods you end up buying, don't feel bad if you end up eating a mix of whole and processed foods. It's okay as long as the ones you pick facilitate your end goal.

Thank you for purchasing this book, I hope you enjoyed it.

Finally, if you enjoyed this book then I'd like to ask you for a favor. Will you be kind enough to leave a review for this book on Amazon? It would be greatly appreciated!

Don't forget to follow us on Twitter, Facebook & Instagram and visit our website www.prosencefitness.com to get empowered, educated and inspired to become the best version of yourself in life! You deserve it.

References

1. Allende, A., Tomas-Barberan, F. A., & Gil, M. I. (2006). Minimal processing for healthy traditional foods. Trends in Food Science & Technology, 17(9), 513-519.

2. Barr, S., & Wright, J. (2010). Postprandial energy expenditure in whole-food and processed-food meals: implications for daily energy expenditure. Food & nutrition research, 54(1), 5144.

3. Bartholomaeus, A., Parrott, W., Bondy, G., Walker, K., & ILSI International Food Biotechnology Committee Task Force on the Use of Mammalian Toxicology Studies in the Safety Assessment of GM Foods. (2013). The use of whole food animal studies in the safety assessment of genetically modified crops: Limitations and recommendations. Critical reviews in toxicology, 43(sup2), 1-24.

4. Batte, M. T., Hooker, N. H., Haab, T. C., & Beaverson, J. (2007). Putting their money where their mouths are: Consumer willingness to pay for multi-ingredient, processed organic food products. Food policy, 32(2), 145-159.

5. Burton-Freeman, B. M., & Sesso, H. D. (2014). Whole food versus supplement: comparing the clinical evidence of tomato intake and lycopene supplementation on cardiovascular risk factors. Advances in Nutrition, 5(5), 457-485.

6. Constable, A., Jonas, D., Cockburn, A., Davi, A., Edwards, G., Hepburn, P., ... & Samuels, F. (2007). History of safe use as applied to the safety assessment of novel foods and foods derived from genetically modified organisms. Food and Chemical Toxicology, 45(12), 2513-2525.

7. Eichler, E. H. (1953). U.S. Patent No. 2,664,358. Washington, DC: U.S. Patent and Trademark Office.

8. Fellows, P. J. (2009). Food processing technology: principles and practice. Elsevier.

9. French, S. A., Story, M., & Jeffery, R. W. (2001). Environmental influences on eating and physical activity. Annual review of public health, 22(1), 309-335.

10. Haff, G., & Triplett, N. T. (2016). Essentials of strength training and conditioning. Champaign, IL: Human Kinetics.

11. Jongwanich, J. (2009). The impact of food safety standards on processed food exports from developing countries. Food Policy, 34(5), 447-457.

12. Lindsay, L. (2000). Credible food safety assurance for the whole meat chain. Nutrition & Food Science, 30(5), 250-253.

13. Liu, R. H. (2003). Health benefits of fruit and vegetables are from additive and synergistic combinations of phytochemicals. The American journal of clinical nutrition, 78(3), 517S-520S.

14. Monteiro, C. A. (2009). Nutrition and health. The issue is not food, nor nutrients, so much as processing. Public health nutrition, 12(5), 729.

15. Monteiro, C. A., Levy, R. B., Claro, R. M., de Castro, I. R. R., & Cannon, G. (2010). Increasing consumption of ultra-processed foods and likely impact on human health: evidence from Brazil. Public health nutrition, 14(1), 5-13.

16. Moubarac, J. C., Martins, A. P. B., Claro, R. M., Levy, R. B., Cannon, G., & Monteiro, C. A. (2013). Consumption of

ultra-processed foods and likely impact on human health. Evidence from Canada. Public Health Nutrition, 16(12), 2240-2248.

17. Oettle, G. J., Emmett, P. M., & Heaton, K. W. (1987). Glucose and insulin responses to manufactured and whole-food snacks. The American journal of clinical nutrition, 45(1), 86-91.

18. Povey, R., Conner, M., Sparks, P., James, R., & Shepherd, R. (1998). Interpretations of healthy and unhealthy eating, and implications for dietary change. Health Education Research, 13(2), 171-183.

19. Ray, K. S., & Singhania, P. R. (2014). Glycemic and insulinemic responses to carbohydrate rich whole foods. Journal of food science and technology, 51(2), 347-352.

20. Mancino, L., Kuchler, F., & Leibtag, E. (2008). Getting consumers to eat more whole-grains: the role of policy, information, and food manufacturers. Food Policy, 33(6), 489-496.

21. Shahidi, F. (2009). Nutraceuticals and functional foods: whole versus processed foods. Trends in Food Science & Technology, 20(9), 376-387.

22. Story, M., Kaphingst, K. M., Robinson-O'Brien, R., & Glanz, K. (2008). Creating healthy food and eating environments: policy and environmental approaches. Annu. Rev. Public Health, 29, 253-272.

23. Weaver, C. M., Dwyer, J., Fulgoni III, V. L., King, J. C., Leveille, G. A., MacDonald, R. S., ... & Schnakenberg, D. (2014). Processed foods: contributions to nutrition. The American journal of clinical nutrition, 99(6), 1525-1542.

www.ingramcontent.com/pod-product-compliance
Lightning Source LLC
Chambersburg PA
CBHW051857250726
48659CB00006B/2260